CU00690412

The Ultimate Plant-Based Diet Cookbook for Beginners

A Beginners Guide to Plant Based Diet Recipes, Very Easy to Prepare for Living and Eating Well Everyday

Virginia Larson

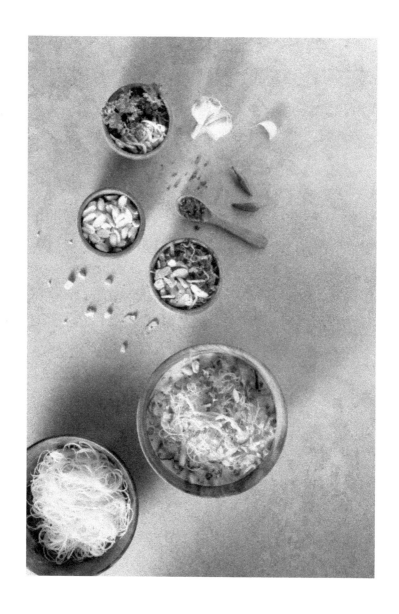

Table of Contents

The information in the following pages is broadly considered a truthful and accurate account of facts and as such, any inattention, use, or misuse of the information in question by the reader will render any resulting actions solely under their purview. There are no scenarios in which the publisher or the original author of this work can be in any fashion deemed liable for any hardship or damages that may befall them after undertaking information described herein.

Additionally, the information in the following pages is intended only for informational purposes and should thus be thought of as universal. As befitting its nature, it is presented without assurance regarding its prolonged validity or interim quality. Trademarks that are mentioned are done without written consent and can in no way be considered an endorsement from the trademark holder.

Introduction

A plant-based diet is a diet based primarily on whole plant foods. It is identical to the regular diet we're used to already, except that it leaves out foods that are not exclusively from plants. Hence, a plant-based diet does away with all types of animal-sourced foods, hydrogenated oils, refined sugars, and processed foods. A whole food plant-based diet comprises not just fruits and vegetables; it also consists of unprocessed or barely-processed oils with healthy monounsaturated fats (like extra-virgin olive oil), whole grains, legumes (essentially lentils and beans), seeds and nuts, as well as herbs and spices.

What makes a plant-based meal (or any meal) fun is the manner with which you make them; the seasoning process; and the combination process that contributes to a fantastic flavor and makes every meal unique and enjoyable. There are lots of delicious recipes (all plant-centered), which will prove helpful in when you intend making mouthwatering, healthy plant-based dishes for personal or household consumption. Provided you're eating these plant-based foods regularly, you'll have very problems with fat or diseases that result from bad dietary habits, and there would be no need for excessive calorie tracking.

Plant-based diet recipes are versatile; they range from colorful Salads to Lentil Stews, and Bean Burritos. The recipes also draw influences from around the globe, with Mexican, Chinese, European, Indian cuisines all part of the vast array of plant-based recipes available to choose from. Why You Ought to Reduce Your Intake of Processed and Animal-Based Foods. You have likely heard over and over that processed food has adverse effects on your health. You might have also been told repeatedly to stay away from foods with lots of preservatives; nevertheless, nobody ever offered any genuine or concrete facts about why you ought to avoid these foods and why they are unsafe. Consequently, let us properly dissect it to help you properly comprehend why you ought to stay away from these healthy eating offenders. They have massive habit-forming characteristics. Humans have a predisposition towards being addicted to some specific foods; however, the reality is that the fault is not wholly ours. Every one of the unhealthy treats we relish now and then triggers the dopamine release in our brains. This creates a pleasurable effect in our brain, but the excitement is usually short-lived. The discharged dopamine additionally causes an attachment connection gradually, and this is the reason some people consistently go back to eat certain unhealthy foods even when they know it's unhealthy and unnecessary.

You can get rid of this by taking out that inducement completely. They are sugar-laden and plenteous in glucose-fructose syrup. Animal-based and processed foods are laden with refined sugars and glucose-fructose syrup which has almost no beneficial food nutrient. An ever-increasing number of studies are affirming what several people presumed from the start; that genetically modified foods bring about inflammatory bowel disease, which consequently makes it increasingly difficult for the body to assimilate essential nutrients. The disadvantages that result from your body being unable to assimilate essential nutrients from consumed foods rightly cannot be overemphasized. Processed and animal-based food products contain plenteous amounts of refined carbohydrates. Indeed, your body requires carbohydrates to give it the needed energy to run body capacities. In any case, refining carbs dispenses with the fundamental supplements; in the way that refining entire grains disposes of the whole grain part. What remains, in the wake of refining, is what's considered as empty carbs or empty calories. These can negatively affect the metabolic system in your body by sharply increasing your blood sugar and insulin quantities. They contain lots of synthetic ingredients. At the point when your body is taking in non-natural ingredients, it regards them as foreign substances.

Your body treats them as a health threat. Your body isn't accustomed to identifying synthetic compounds like sucralose or these synthesized sugars. Hence, in defense of your health against this foreign "aggressor," your body does what it's capable of to safeguard your health. It sets off an immune reaction to tackle this "enemy" compound, which indirectly weakens your body's general disease alertness, making you susceptible to illnesses. The concentration and energy expended by your body in ensuring your immune system remain safe could instead be devoted somewhere else. They contain constituent elements that set off an excitable reward sensation in your body. A part of processed and animal-based foods contain compounds like glucose-fructose syrup, monosodium glutamate, and specific food dyes that can trigger some addiction. They rouse your body to receive a benefit in return whenever you consume them. Monosodium glutamate, for example, is added to many store-bought baked foods. This additive slowly conditions your palates to relish the taste. It gets mental just by how your brain interrelates with your taste sensors.

This reward-centric arrangement makes you crave it increasingly, which ends up exposing you to the danger of over consuming calories.

For animal protein, usually, the expression "subpar" is used to allude to plant proteins since they generally have lower levels of essential amino acids as against animal-sourced protein. Nevertheless, what the vast majority don't know is that large amounts of essential amino acids can prove detrimental to your health. Let me break it down further for you.

Farro and Lentil Salad

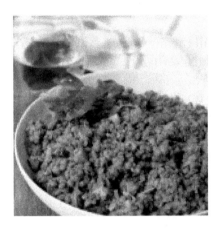

Preparation Time: 10 minutes
Cooking Time: 0 minutes
Servings: 4
Ingredients:
For the Salad:

      1 cup grape tomato, halved
      ½ cup diced yellow bell pepper
      1 cup diced cucumber,
      ½ cup diced red bell pepper
      1 cup fresh arugula
      1/3 cup chopped parsley
      1 ½ cups lentils, cooked
      3 ½ cups farro, cooked

For the Dressing:

      ½ teaspoon minced garlic
      ½ teaspoon salt
      ¼ teaspoon ground black pepper
      1 teaspoon Italian seasoning
      1 teaspoon Dijon mustard
      2 tablespoons red wine vinegar

2 tablespoons lemon juice
1/3 cup olive oil

Directions:

Take a large bowl, place all the ingredients for the salad in it except for arugula and then toss until combined.

Prepare the dressing and for this, take a medium bowl, add all of its ingredients in it and then stir whisk until well combined.

Pour the dressing over the salad, toss until well coated, then distribute salad among four bowls and top with arugula.

Serve straight away.

Nutrition:

379 Cal
10 g Fat
2 g Saturated Fat
63.5 g Carbohydrates
11 g Fiber
2.5 g Sugars
12.5 g Protein;

Greek Zoodle Bowl

Preparation Time: 10 minutes
Cooking Time: 0 minutes
Servings: 4
Ingredients:

½ cup chopped artichokes
14 cherry tomatoes, chopped
1 medium red bell peppers, cored, chopped
4 medium zucchini
1 medium yellow bell pepper, cored, chopped
6 tablespoons hemp hearts
1 English cucumber
6 tablespoons chopped red onion
2 tablespoons chopped parsley leaves
2 tablespoons chopped mint

For the Greek Dressing:

2 tablespoons chopped mint
1 teaspoon garlic powder
½ teaspoon salt
¼ teaspoon dried oregano
2 teaspoons Italian seasoning
3 tablespoons red wine vinegar
1 tablespoon olive oil

Directions:

Prepare zucchini and cucumber noodles and for this, spiralize them by using a spiralizer or vegetable peeler and then divide evenly among four bowls.

Top zucchini and cucumber noodles with artichokes, tomato, bell pepper, hemp hearts, onion, parsley, and mint and then set aside until required.

Prepare the dressing and for this, take a small bowl, add all the ingredients for the dressing in it and whisk until combined.

Add the prepared dressing evenly into each bowl, then toss until the vegetables are well coated with the dressing and serve.

Nutrition:
250 Cal
14 g Fat
3 g Saturated Fat
19 g Carbohydrates
5 g Fiber
9 g Sugars
13 g Protein;

Roasted Vegetables and Quinoa Bowls

Preparation Time: 10 minutes
Cooking Time: 20 minutes
Servings: 4
Ingredients:

3 cups cooked quinoa

For the Broccoli:

2 teaspoons minced garlic
4 cups broccoli florets
½ teaspoon salt
¼ teaspoon ground black pepper
4 teaspoons olive oil

For the Chickpeas:

4 teaspoons sriracha
3 cups cooked chickpeas
2 teaspoons olive oil
4 teaspoons soy sauce

For the Roasted Sweet Potatoes:

2 teaspoons curry powder
2 small sweet potatoes, peeled, ¼-inch thick sliced
1/8 teaspoon salt
2 teaspoons sriracha
2 teaspoons olive oil

For the Chili-Lime Kale:

1/2 of a lime, juiced
4 cups chopped kale
1/8 teaspoon salt
1/8 teaspoon ground black pepper
1 teaspoon red chili powder
2 teaspoons olive oil

Directions:

Switch on the oven, then set it to 400 degrees F and let it preheat.

Prepare broccoli florets and for this, take a large bowl, place all of its ingredients in it, toss until well coated, then take a baking sheet lined with parchment paper and spread florets in a one-third portion of the sheet in a row.

Add chickpeas into the bowl, add its remaining ingredients, toss until well mixed and spread them onto the baking sheet next to the broccoli florets.

Add sweet potatoes into the bowl, add its remaining ingredients, toss until well mixed and spread them onto the baking sheet next to the chickpeas.

Place the baking sheet containing vegetables and chickpeas into the oven and then bake for 20 minutes until vegetables have turned tender and chickpeas are slightly crispy, turning halfway.

Meanwhile, prepare the kale and for this, take a large skillet pan, place it over medium heat, add 1 teaspoon oil and when hot, add kale and cook for 5 minutes until tender.

Then season kale with salt, black pepper, and red chili powder, toss until mixed and continue cooking for 3 minutes, set aside until required.

Assemble the bowl and for this, distribute quinoa evenly among four bowls, top evenly with broccoli, chickpeas, sweet potatoes, and kale and then serve.

Nutrition:

415 Cal
17 g Fat
2 g Saturated Fat
54 g Carbohydrates
8 g Fiber
5 g Sugars
16 g Protein;

Sweet Potato and Quinoa Bowl

Preparation Time: 5 minutes
Cooking Time: 20 minutes
Servings: 4
Ingredients:

>   2 cups quinoa
>   1 cup diced red onion
>   2 cups diced sweet potato
>   1 1/2 cup raisins
>   1 cup sunflower seeds, shelled, unsalted
>   2 cups vegetable broth

Directions:

>   Take a medium pot, place it over high heat, add quinoa, and sweet potatoes, pour in vegetable broth, stir until mixed and bring it to a boil.
>   Then switch heat to medium-low level, cover pot with the lid, and cook for 20 minutes until the quinoa has cooked.
>   When done, remove the pot from heat and fluff quinoa by using a fork.
>   Add onion, raisins, and sunflower seeds, stir until mixed and transfer into a large bowl.
>   Let it chill in the refrigerator for 30 minutes and then serve.

Nutrition:
204 Cal
7 g Fat
3 g Saturated Fat
31 g Carbohydrates
3 g Fiber
11 g Sugars
3 g Protein;

Chickpea Salad Bites

Preparation Time: 15 minutes
Cooking Time: 0 minutes
Servings: 4
Ingredients:
For the Bread:

> 2 tablespoons chopped parsley
> 1 small green chili pepper
> 1/3 cup of raisins
> 1 teaspoon garlic powder
> ½ teaspoon salt
> 1/3 teaspoon ground black pepper
> ½ teaspoon smoked paprika
> ½ tablespoon maple syrup
> ½ teaspoon cayenne pepper
> 2 tablespoons balsamic vinegar
> 1 1/2 cups crumbled rye bread, whole-grain

For the Salad:

> 2 scallions, chopped
> 1/3 cup chopped pickles
> 2 tablespoons chopped chives and more for topping
> ½ teaspoon minced garlic
> 1 ½ cup cooked chickpeas
> 1 lemon, juiced
> ½ teaspoon salt
> ¼ teaspoon ground black pepper
> 1 tablespoons poppy seeds
> 1 teaspoon mustard paste
> 1/3 cup coconut yogurt

Directions:

> Prepare the bread, and for this, place all of its ingredients in a food processor and then pulse for 1 minute until just combined; don't over mix.

Then make bites of the bread mixture and for this, take a 2.3-inch round cookie cutter, add 2 tablespoons of the bread mixture, press it into the cutter, and gently lift it out, repeat with the remaining batter to make seven more bites.

Prepare the salad and for this, take a large bowl, add chickpeas in it, then add chives, scallion, pickles, and garlic and then mash chickpeas by using a fork until broken.

Add remaining ingredients for the salad and stir until well mixed.

Assemble the bites and for this, top each prepared bread bite generously with prepared salad, sprinkle with chives and poppy seeds, and then serve.

Nutrition:
210 Cal
4 g Fat
1 g Saturated Fat
36 g Carbohydrates
6 g Fiber
4 g Sugars
7 g Protein;

Avocado and Chickpeas Lettuce Cups

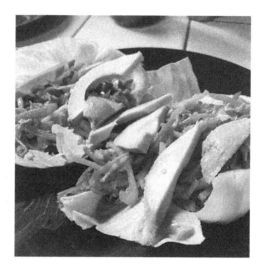

Preparation Time: 10 minutes
Cooking Time: 0 minutes
Servings: 4
Ingredients:

  2 small avocados, peeled, pitted, diced
  8 ounces hearts of palm
  ¾ cup cooked chickpeas
  1/2 cup cucumber, diced
  1 tablespoon minced shallots
  2 cups mixed greens
  1 tablespoon Dijon mustard
  1 lime, zested, juiced
  2 tablespoons chopped cilantro and more for topping
  2/3 teaspoon salt
  1/3 teaspoon ground black pepper
  1 tablespoon apple cider vinegar
  2 ½ tablespoons olive oil

Directions:

Take a medium bowl, add shallots and cilantro in it, stir in salt, black pepper, mustard, vinegar, lime juice, and zest until just mixed and then slowly mix in olive oil until combined.

Add cucumber, hearts of palm and chickpeas, stir until mixed, fold in avocado and then top with some more cilantro.

Distribute mixed greens among four plates, top with chickpea mixture and then serve.

Nutrition:
280 Cal
12.6 g Fat
1.5 g Saturated Fat
32.8 g Carbohydrates
9.3 g Fiber
1.2 g Sugars - 7.6 g Protein

Pesto Quinoa with White Beans

Preparation Time: 5 minutes
Cooking Time: 15 minutes
Servings: 4
Ingredients:

12 ounces cooked white bean
3 ½ cups quinoa, cooked
1 medium zucchini, sliced
¾ cup sun-dried tomato
¼ cup pine nuts
1 tablespoon olive oil

For the Pesto:

1/3 cup walnuts
2 cups arugula
1 teaspoon minced garlic
2 cups basil
¾ teaspoon salt
¼ teaspoon ground black pepper
1 tablespoon lemon juice
1/3 cup olive oil
2 tablespoons water

Directions:

Prepare the pesto, and for this, place all of its
ingredients in a food processor and pulse for 2
minutes until smooth, scraping the sides of the
container frequently and set aside until required.
Take a large skillet pan, place it over medium heat, add
oil and when hot, add zucchini and cook for 4
minutes until tender-crisp.
Season zucchini with salt and black pepper, cook for 2
minutes until lightly brown, then add tomatoes and
white beans and continue cooking for 4 minutes
until white beans begin to crisp.

Stir in pine nuts, cook for 2 minutes until toasted, then remove the pan from heat and transfer zucchini mixture into a medium bowl.

Add quinoa and pesto, stir until well combined, then distribute among four bowls and then serve.

Nutrition:

352 Cal
27.3 g Fat
5 g Saturated Fat
33.7 g Carbohydrates
5.7 g Fiber
4.5 g Sugars
9.7 g Protein;

Pumpkin Risotto

Preparation Time: 5 minutes
Cooking Time: 20 minutes
Servings: 4
Ingredients:

1 cup Arborio rice
½ cup cooked and chopped pumpkin
1/2 cup mushrooms
1 rib of celery, diced
½ of a medium white onion, peeled, diced
½ teaspoon minced garlic
½ teaspoon salt
1/3 teaspoon ground black pepper
1 tablespoon olive oil
½ tablespoon coconut butter
1 cup pumpkin puree
2 cups vegetable stock

Directions:

Take a medium saucepan, place it over medium heat, add oil and when hot, add onion and celery, stir in garlic and cook for 3 minutes until onions begin to soften.

Add mushrooms, season with salt and black pepper and cook for 5 minutes.

Add rice, pour in pumpkin puree, then gradually pour in the stock until rice soaked up all the liquid and have turned soft.

Add butter, remove the pan from heat, stir until creamy mixture comes together, and then serve.

Nutrition:
218.5 Cal
5.2 g Fat
1.5 g Saturated Fat
32.3 g Carbohydrates
1.3 g Fiber - 3.8 g Sugars - 6.3 g Protein;

Brown Rice and Vegetable Stir-Fry

Preparation Time: 5 minutes
Cooking Time: 50 minutes
Servings: 4
Ingredients:

- 16-ounce tofu, extra-firm, pressed, drained, cut into ½-inch cubes
- 1 cup of brown rice
- 1 cup frozen broccoli florets
- 1 medium red bell pepper, cored, diced
- 1 small white onion, peeled, diced
- 1 tablespoon minced garlic
- ½ teaspoon salt
- 1/3 teaspoon ground black pepper
- 1 tablespoon olive oil
- 2 cups vegetable broth

Directions:

Take a medium pot, place it over high heat, add brown rice, pour in vegetable broth, and bring it to a boil.

Switch heat to medium-low level, cover the pot with the lid and cook for 40 minutes, and when done, remove the pot and set aside until required.

Then take a large skillet pan, place it over medium-high heat, add oil and when hot, add tofu pieces, onion, broccoli, and bell pepper, season with salt and black pepper and cook for 5 minutes until sauté.

Add cooked rice, stir until mixed and continue cooking for 5 minutes.

Serve straight away.

Nutrition:

281.9 Cal
11.7 g Fat
1.7 g Saturated Fat
31.1 g Carbohydrates
9.7 g Fiber - 2.1 g Sugars - 20.1 g Protein;

Tomato Basil Spaghetti

Preparation Time: 5 minutes
Cooking Time: 20 minutes
Servings: 4
Ingredients:

>15-ounce cooked great northern beans
>10.5-ounces cherry tomatoes, halved
>1 small white onion, peeled, diced
>1 tablespoon minced garlic
>8 basil leaves, chopped
>2 tablespoons olive oil
>1-pound spaghetti

Directions:

>Take a large pot half full with salty water, place it over medium-high heat, bring it to a boil, add spaghetti and cook for 10 to 12 minutes until tender.
>Then drain spaghetti into a colander and reserve 1 cup of pasta liquid.
>Take a large skillet pan, place it over medium-high heat, add oil and when hot, add onion, tomatoes, basil, and garlic and cook for 5 minutes until vegetables have turned tender.
>Add cooked spaghetti and beans, pour in pasta water, stir until just mixed and cook for 2 minutes until hot.
>Serve straight away.

Nutrition:

147 Cal
5 g Fat
0.7 g Saturated Fat
21.2 g Carbohydrates
1.5 g Fiber
5.4 g Sugars
3.8 g Protein;

Jamaican Jerk Tofu Wrap

Preparation Time: 1 hour and 15 minutes
Cooking Time: 16 minutes
Servings: 4
Ingredients:

28 ounces tofu, firmed, pressed, drain, ½-inch long sliced

For the Marinade:

2 small scotch bonnet pepper, deseeded, minced
2 teaspoons minced garlic
2 1/2 teaspoons sea salt
4 teaspoons allspice
2 teaspoon ground black pepper
4 teaspoons cinnamon
4 teaspoons maple syrup
4 teaspoons nutmeg
4 tablespoons apple cider vinegar
2 teaspoon avocado oil and more for cooking
½ cup of soy sauce
2 tablespoon tomato paste

For the Wrap:

4 cups baby spinach leaves
2 small tomato, deseeded, diced
2 medium yellow bell pepper, deseeded, cut into strips
4 tablespoons Sriracha sauce
4 tortillas, whole-grain

Directions:

Take a large bowl, place all the ingredients for the marinade in it, whisk until combined, then add tofu pieces, toss until well coated, and let it marinate for a minimum of 1 hour, turning halfway.

Then take a large skillet pan, place it over medium-high heat, add some of the avocado oil, and when hot, add tofu pieces in a single layer and cook for 8 minutes per side until caramelized.

Assemble the wrap and for this, place a tortilla on clean working space, top with 1 cup of spinach, half of each diced tomatoes and pepper strips, then top with 4 strips of tofu, drizzle with Sriracha sauce and wrap tightly.

Repeat with the remaining tortilla, then cut each tortilla in half and serve.

Nutrition:
250 Cal
6 g Fat
1 g Saturated Fat
40 g Carbohydrates
7 g Fiber
11 g Sugars
9 g Protein;

Chickpea Curry Soup

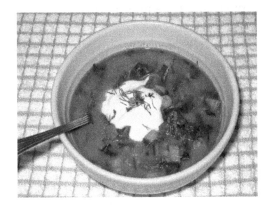

Preparation Time: 5 minutes
Cooking Time: 12 minutes
Servings: 4
Ingredients:

> 2 cups cooked chickpeas
> 1/4 of a medium white onion, peeled, chopped
> 1 tablespoon minced garlic
> 1 teaspoon ground coriander
> ¼ teaspoon cayenne pepper
> 1 tablespoon yellow curry powder
> 1 teaspoon turmeric
> ½ of a lime, juiced
> 1 tablespoon olive oil
> 2/3 cup coconut cream
> 2 cups vegetable broth
> 2 tablespoons pumpkin seeds

Directions:

> Take a medium saucepan, place it over medium-high
> heat, add oil and when hot, add onion and garlic
> and cook for 1 minute until fragrant.

Add chickpeas, sprinkle with all the spices, stir until
mixed and continue cooking for 5 minutes.

Pour in vegetable broth, simmer for 5 minutes, then
stir in cream, lime juice and remove the pan from
heat.

Ladle soup into bowls, top with pumpkin seeds, and
then serve.

Nutrition:
154 Cal
8 g Fat
1 g Saturated Fat
16.5 g Carbohydrates
4 g Fiber
3 g Sugars
4.5 g Protein;

Sweet Potato Sushi

Preparation Time: 90 minutes

Cooking Time: 35 minutes

Serving: 3

Ingredients:

- 1 14-oz. package silken tofu, drained
- 3 nori sheets
- 1 large sweet potato, peeled
- 1 medium avocado, pitted, peeled, sliced
- 1 cup water
- ¾ cup dry sushi rice
- 1 tbsp. rice vinegar
- 1 tbsp. agave nectar
- 1 tbsp. amino acids

Directions:

1. Preheat the oven to 400°F / 200°C.

2. Stir the amino acids (or tamari) and agave nectar together in a small bowl until it is well combined and set aside.

3. Cut the sweet potato into large sticks, around ½-inch thick. Place them on a baking sheet lined with parchment and coat them with the tamari/agave mixture.

4. Bake the sweet potatoes in the oven until softened—for about 25 minutes—and make sure to flip them halfway so the sides cook evenly.

5. Meanwhile, bring the sushi rice, water, and vinegar to a boil in a medium-sized pot over medium heat, and cook until liquid has evaporated, for about 10 minutes.

6. While cooking the rice, cut the block of tofu into long sticks. The sticks should look like long, thin fries. Set aside.

7. Remove the pot from heat and let the rice sit for 10-15 minutes.

8. Cover your work area with a piece of parchment paper, clean your hands, wet your fingers, and lay out a sheet of nori on the parchment paper.

9. Cover the nori sheet with a thin layer of sushi rice, while wetting the hands frequently. Leave sufficient space for rolling up the sheet.

10. Place the roasted sweet potato strips in a straight line across the width of the sheet, about an inch away from the edge closest to you.

11. Lay out the tofu and avocado slices right beside the potato sticks and use the parchment paper as an aid to roll up the nori sheet into a tight cylinder.

12. Slice the cylinder into 8 equal pieces and refrigerate. Repeat the process for the remaining nori sheets and fillings.

13. Serve chilled, or, store to enjoy this delicious sushi later!

Nutrition:

Calories 467, Total Fat 17.1g, Saturated Fat 3.4g, Cholesterol 0mg, Sodium 81mg, Total Carbohydrate 64g, Dietary Fiber 7.6g, Total Sugars 11g, Protein 15.4g, Vitamin D 0mcg, Calcium 78mg, Iron 6mg, Potassium 921mg

Bean and Rice Burritos

Preparation Time: 10 minutes
Cooking Time: 20 minutes
Servings: 6
Ingredients:

32 ounces refried beans
2 cups cooked rice
2 cups chopped spinach
1 tablespoon olive oil
1/2 cup tomato salsa
6 tortillas, whole-grain, warm
Guacamole as needed for serving

Directions:

Switch on the oven, then set it to 375 degrees F and let it preheat.

Take a medium saucepan, place it over medium heat, add beans, and cook for 3 to 5 minutes until softened, remove the pan from heat.

Place one tortilla on clean working space, spread some of the beans on it into a log, leaving 2-inches of the edge, top beans with spinach, rice and salsa, and then tightly wrap the tortilla to seal the filling like a burrito.

Repeat with the remaining tortillas, place these burritos on a baking sheet, brush them with olive oil and then bake for 15 minutes until golden.

Serve burritos with guacamole.

Nutrition:
421 Cal
9 g Fat
2 g Saturated Fat
70 g Carbohydrates
11 g Fiber
3 g Sugars
15 g Protein;

Fast Twitch Quinoa

Preparation Time: 5 minutes

Cooking Time: 0 minute

Serving: 7

Ingredients

- 3 tablespoons olive oil
- Juice of 1½ lemons
- 1 teaspoon garlic powder
- ½ teaspoon dried oregano
- 1 bunch curly kale
- 2 cups cooked tricolor quinoa
- 1 cup canned mandarin oranges in juice
- 1 cup diced yellow summer squash
- 1 red bell pepper
- ½ red onion
- ½ cup dried cranberries
- ½ cup slivered almonds

Direction

1. Scourge the oil, lemon juice, garlic powder, and oregano.
2. Mix the kale with the oil-lemon mixture until well coated. Add the quinoa, oranges, squash, bell pepper, and red onion and toss until all the ingredients are well combined. Divide among

bowls or transfer to a large serving platter. Top with the cranberries and almonds.

Nutrition:

343 Calories

24g Protein

11g Fiber

Tuna Cakes

Preparation Time: 5 minutes
Cooking Time: 6 minutes
Servings: 2
Ingredients:

> 5-ounce tuna, packed in water
> 1 tablespoon mustard
> 1 teaspoon garlic powder
> 1 tablespoon coconut oil

Extra:

> ¼ teaspoon salt
> 1/8 teaspoon ground black pepper

Directions:

> Drain the tuna, add it in a medium bowl and break it well with a fork.
> Then add remaining ingredients, stir until well mixed and then shape the mixture into four patties.
> Take a medium skillet pan, place it over medium heat, add oil and when hot, add tuna patties and cook for 3 minutes per side until golden brown.
> Serve patties straight away or serve as a wrap with iceberg lettuce.

Nutrition:
Calories 115
Fat 9
Carbs 12
Protein 4

Spicy Root and Lentil Casserole

Preparation Time: 10 minutes

Cooking Time: 35 minutes

Serving: 4

Ingredients:

- 2 tbsp vegetable oil
- 1 onion, chopped
- 2 garlic cloves, crushed
- 700g potatoes, peeled and cut into chunks
- 4 carrot, thickly sliced
- 2 parsnip, thickly sliced
- 2 tbsp curry paste or powder
- 1 liter/1¾ pints vegetable stock
- 100g red lentils

Direction

1. Cook oil in a large pan, cook the onion and garlic over a medium heat for 3 minutes. Continue stirring in between to cook them well. Add potatoes, carrots and parsnips, turn up the heat and cook for 6 to 7 minutes. Stir well

2. Stir in the curry paste or powder, fill in the stock, and bring to a boil. Reduce the heat, add the lentils. Cover and simmer for 18 minutes.

3. Once done, season with coriander and heat for a minute. Serve with yogurt and the rest of the coriander.

Nutrition:

378 Calories

14g Protein

10g Fiber

Seitan

Preparation Time: 25 minutes

Cooking Time: 20 minutes

Serving: 5

Ingredients

- Firm Tofu, 250 grams
- Unsweetened soy milk, 150ml
- Miso paste 2 tsp
- Marmite 2 tsp
- Onion powder 1 tsp
- Garlic powder 2 tsp
- Wheat gluten 160g
- Pea protein or vegan protein powder, 40g
- Vegetable stock 1 ½ liters

Direction

1. Blitz the tofu, soy milk, miso, marmite, onion powder, garlic powder, 1 tsp salt and ½ tsp white pepper in a food processor. Blend until smooth.
2. Mix them all to form a dough. Knead the dough well, stretching and tearing for 10-15 minutes.
3. Fill vegetable stock into a pan and let it simmer. Flatten out the seitan to a thickness of 1 cm and

chop into chunks. Simmer it in the stock for 20 minutes covering with a lid. Once it's done, allow it to cool down. Chop or tear it into smaller pieces before cooking as per your choice.

Nutrition:

211Calories

35g Protein

2g Fiber

Vegan Alfredo Fettuccine Pasta

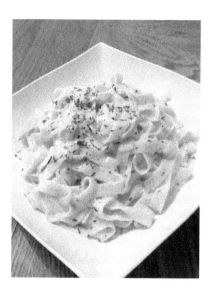

Preparation Time: 15 minutes
Cooking Time: 15 minutes
Servings: 1
Ingredients:

> White potatoes - 2 medium
> White onion - ¼
> Italian seasoning - 1 tablespoon
> Lemon juice - 1 teaspoon
> Garlic - 2 cloves
> Salt - 1 teaspoon
> Fettuccine pasta - 12 ounces
> Raw cashew - ½ cup
> Nutritional yeast (optional) - 1 teaspoon
> Truffle oil (optional) - ¼ teaspoon

Directions:

> Start by placing a pot on high flame and boiling 4 cups
> of water.

Peel the potatoes and cut them into small cubes. Cut the onion into cubes as well.

Add the potatoes and onions to the boiling water and cook for about 10 minutes.

Remove the onions and potatoes. Keep aside. Save the water.

Take another pot and fill it with water. Season generously with salt.

Toss in the fettuccine pasta and cook as per package instructions.

Take a blender and add in the raw cashews, veggies, nutritional yeast, truffle oil, lemon juice, and 1 cup of the saved water. Blend into a smooth puree.

Add in the garlic and salt.

Drain the cooked pasta using a colander. Transfer into a mixing bowl.

Pour the prepared sauce on top of the cooked fettuccine pasta. Serve.

Nutrition:
Calories 884
Fat 13
Carbs 15
Protein 6

Spinach Pasta in Pesto Sauce

Preparation Time: 20 minutes
Cooking Time: 15 minutes
Servings: 1
Ingredients:

    Olive oil - 1 tablespoon
    Spinach - 5 ounces
    All-purpose flour - 2 cups
    Salt - 1 tablespoon plus ¼ teaspoon (keep it divided)
    Water - 2 tablespoons
    Roasted vegetable for serving
    Pesto for serving
    Fresh basil for serving

Directions:

Take a large pot and fill it with water. Place it over a high flame and bring the water to a boil. Add one tablespoon of salt

While the water is boiling, place a large saucepan over medium flame. Pour in the olive oil and heat it through.

Once the oil starts to shimmer, toss in the spinach and sauté for 5 minutes.

Take a food processor and transfer the wilted spinach. Process until the spinach is fine in texture.

Add in the flour bit by bit and continue to process to form a crumbly dough.

Further, add ¼ teaspoon of salt and 1 tbsp of water while processing to bring the dough together. Add the remaining 1 tbsp of water if required.

Remove the dough onto a flat surface and sprinkle with flour. Knead well to form a dough ball.

Use a rolling pin to roll out the dough. The dimensions of the rolled dough should be 18 inches long and 12 inches wide. The thickness should be about ¼ - inch thick.

Cut the rolled dough into long and even strips using a pizza cutter. Make sure the strips are ½ - inch wide.

The strips need to be rolled into evenly sized thick noodles.

Toss in the prepared noodles and cook for about 4 minutes. Drain using a colander.

Transfer the noodles into a large mixing bowl and add in the roasted vegetables, pesto. Toss well to combine.

Garnish with basil leaves.

Nutrition:
Calories 591
Fat 8
Carbs 42
Protein 16

Mushroom Zucchini Pasta

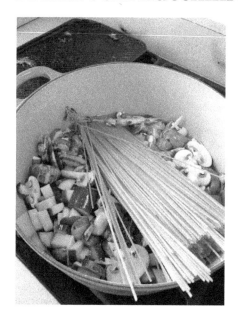

Preparation Time: 8 min.

Cooking Time: 20 min.

Servings: *5-6*

Ingredients:

- 12 mushrooms, thinly sliced
- 1 zucchini, thinly sliced
- A few drops of sherry wine
- 1 shallot, finely chopped
- 15 ounces penne pasta
- 5 ounces tomato paste
- 2 tablespoons soy sauce

- 1 yellow onion, thinly sliced
- 2 garlic cloves, minced
- 1 tablespoon olive oil
- 1 cup vegetable stock
- 2 cups water
- A pinch of basil, dried
- A pinch of oregano, dried
- Black pepper and salt as needed

Directions:

1. Take your Instant Pot and place it on a clean kitchen platform. Turn it on after plugging it into a power socket.
2. Put the pot on "Saute" mode. In the pot, add the oil, onion, shallot, pepper and salt; cook for 2-3 minutes until the ingredients become soft.
3. Add the garlic, stir and cook for 1 minute more. Mix in the mushrooms, zucchini, basil, and oregano, stir and cook 1 more minute.
4. Mix in the wine, stock, water and soy sauce; stir well and then add the pasta and tomato sauce. Add more pepper and salt, if needed.
5. Close the lid and lock. Ensure that you have sealed the valve to avoid leakage.

6. Press "Manual" mode and set timer for 5 minutes. It will take a few minutes for the pot to build inside pressure and start cooking.
7. After the timer reads zero, press "Cancel" and quick release pressure.
8. Carefully remove the lid and serve warm!

Nutrition:

Calories - 248

Fat – 12.5g

Carbohydrates – 12g

Fiber – 1g

Protein – 3.5g

Gear Up Lentils

Preparation Time: 5 minutes

Cooking Time: 40 minutes

Serving: 6

Ingredients

- 5 cups water
- 2¼ cups brown lentils
- 3 teaspoons minced garlic
- 1 bay leaf
- ½ teaspoon dried basil
- ½ teaspoon dried oregano
- ½ teaspoon dried rosemary
- ½ teaspoon dried thyme

Direction:

1. Boil water, lentils, garlic, bay leaf, basil, oregano, rosemary, and thyme. Decrease heat to low, and simmer for 35 minutes. Drain any excess cooking liquid.
2. Transfer to a container, or scoop 1 cup of lentils into each of 6 storage containers. Let cool before sealing the lids.

Nutrition: 257 Calories - 1g Fat - 19g Protein

Creamy Curry Noodles

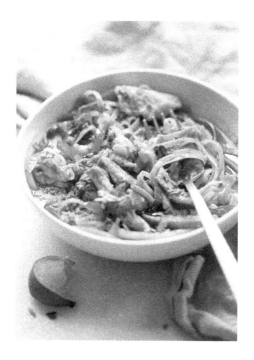

Preparation Time: 19 minutes
Cooking Time: 10 minutes
Servings: 4
Ingredients:
Creamy Curry Sauce

      Apple cider vinegar, two tablespoons
      Water, one-quarter of one cup
      Avocado oil, two tablespoons
      Turmeric, ground, one teaspoon
      Black pepper, one half teaspoon
      Tahini, one-quarter of one cup
      Coriander, ground, one- and one-half teaspoons
      Cumin, ground, one teaspoon
      Salt, one teaspoon

Curry powder, two teaspoons
Ginger, ground, one quarter teaspoon

Noodle Bowl

Cilantro, fresh, chopped small, one half cup
Bell pepper, red, one cleaned and diced
Zucchini noodles, one sixteen-ounce pack
Carrots, two, peeled and cut in julienne strips
Kale, two cups packed
Cauliflower, one half of one head chopped small

Directions:

Cover the zucchini noodles with two cups of boiling water in a medium-sized bowl and set them off to the side. After leaving the noodles in the water for five minutes, drain off the water and place the noodles back into the bowl. Prep all of the veggies and then toss them into the bowl with the noodles. Toss the ingredients in the bowl gently, but well.

Divide the leaves of kale onto four serving plates. Mix the list of ingredients for the Creamy Curry Sauce and blend them until they are smooth and creamy. When the sauce is well mixed, then pour it over the ingredients in the bowl and toss the ingredients well until all are covered with the sauce.

Then divide the noodles over the kale on the four plates and serve.

Nutrition:
Calories 192
Fat 15
Carbs 5
Protein 8

Roasted Vegetables

Preparation Time: 10 minutes
Cooking Time: 20 minutes
Servings: 4
Ingredients:

>Cilantro, chopped, one-quarter of one cup
>Green onion, diced, one half of one cup

Masala Seasoning

>Black pepper, one half teaspoon
>Turmeric, one quarter teaspoon
>Chili powder, ground, one half teaspoon
>Tomato puree, one half of one cup
>Garam masala, one quarter teaspoon
>Salt, one half teaspoon
>Garlic, minced, one tablespoon
>Olive oil, two tablespoons
>Ginger, ground, two teaspoons

Veggies

>Cauliflower, one cup in small pieces
>Mushrooms, sliced one half of one cup
>Green beans, three-fourths of one cup

Directions:

>Heat the oven to 400. Place the rack in the oven in the middle. Use aluminum foil or parchment paper to completely cover a baking sheet. Chop the veggies if they are not already chopped. Use a medium-sized bowl to mix the chili powder, ginger, garam masala, garlic, pepper, salt, and the tomato puree, making sure the ingredients are all mixed well.
>Then mix in the olive oil. Place the chopped veggies into this mixture and mix them in well. Then place the coated veggies onto the covered baking sheet in one single layer.

Roast the veggies in the heated oven for thirty to forty minutes or until the veggies are cooked in a manner in which you like them.

Nutrition:
Calories 105
Fat 10
Carbs 13
Protein 3

Green Pea Fritter

Preparation Time: 10 minutes
Cooking Time: 20 minutes
Servings: 10
Ingredients:

Frozen peas, two cups
Olive oil, one tablespoon + one tablespoon
Onion, one diced
Garlic, three tablespoons
Chickpea four, one- and one-half cups
Baking soda, one teaspoon
Salt, one quarter teaspoon
Rosemary, one teaspoon
Thyme, one half teaspoon
Marjoram, one teaspoon
Lemon juice, two tablespoons

Directions:

Heat the oven to 350. Use spray oil to spray a baking sheet. Boil the peas for five minutes.

Pour one tablespoon of olive oil in a skillet and fry the garlic and onion for five minutes.

Pour the garlic and onion with the olive oil in a bowl and add the cooked peas, mashing them until they make a thick paste. Blend in the marjoram, thyme, rosemary, salt, baking soda, and chickpea flour.

Dampen your hands and form the mash into ten equal-sized patties. Brush the patties with the other tablespoon of olive oil.

Bake them for eighteen minutes in the oven, turning them over after nine minutes.

Nutrition:

Calories 224
Fat 3
Carbs 14
Protein 6

Roasted Mushrooms and Shallots

Preparation Time: 10 minutes
Cooking Time: 20 minutes
Servings: 4
Ingredients:

Mushrooms, fresh, one-pound cut into bite-size pieces
Shallots, two cups sliced thick
Olive oil, two tablespoons
Thyme, dried, one teaspoon
Salt, one quarter teaspoon
Black pepper, one quarter teaspoon
Red wine vinegar, one third cup

Directions:

Heat your oven to 450.

Place the shallots and mushrooms in a large bowl and add in the salt, pepper, thyme, and olive oil and toss the ingredients together to thoroughly coat the shallots and mushrooms.

Roast the veggies on a baking sheet for fifteen minutes. Pour the red wine vinegar over the veggies and bake for five more minutes.

Nutrition:

Calories 178
Fat 7
Carbs 23
Protein 5

Garlic Chili Roasted Kohlrabi

Preparation Time: 5 minutes
Cooking Time: 12 minutes
Servings: 1
Ingredients:

> Olive oil, two tablespoons
> Garlic, minced, one tablespoon
> Chili pepper, one teaspoon
> Salt, one quarter teaspoon
> Kohlrabi, one and one-half pounds, peel and cut into
> one half inch wedges
> Cilantro, fresh, chopped, two tablespoons

Directions:

> Heat your oven to 450. Mix in a large bowl, the pepper,
> salt, chili pepper, garlic, and olive oil. Put in the
> kohlrabi and toss well to coat the kohlrabi.
> Bake the coated kohlrabi for twenty minutes, stirring it
> around when you are about halfway done with
> cooking. Sprinkle on the cilantro and serve.

Nutrition:

Calories 185
Fat 5
Carbs 7
Protein 3

Vegetarian Nachos

Preparation Time: 15 minutes
Cooking Time: 0 minutes
Servings: 6
Ingredients:

Pita chips, whole wheat, three cups
Nutritional yeast, one half cup
Oregano, dried, one tablespoon minced
Romaine lettuce, one cup chopped
Grape tomatoes, one-half cup cut in quarters
Olive oil, two tablespoons
Lemon juice, one tablespoon
Hummus, one-third cup prepared
Black pepper, one half teaspoon
Red onion, two tablespoons minced
Tofu, one-half cup cut into small crumbles
Black olives, two tablespoons chopped

Directions:

Mix the hummus, pepper, olive oil, and lemon juice in
a mixing bowl. Spread a layer of the pita chips on a
serving platter.

Drizzle three-fourths of the hummus mix over the pita
chips. Use the lettuce, red onion, tomatoes, and
olives to garnish the hummus.

Make a small mound of the leftover hummus in the
middle of the chips, then garnish all with the
oregano and the nutritional yeast.

Nutrition:

Calories 159
Fat 10
Carbs 13
Protein 4

Ruby Red Root Beet Burger

Preparation Time: 20 minutes

Cooking Time: 21 minutes

Serving: 6

Ingredients:

- 1 cup dry chickpeas
- ½ cup dry quinoa
- 2 large beets
- 2 tbsp. olive oil
- 2 tbsp. garlic powder
- 1 tbsp. balsamic vinegar
- 2 tsp. onion powder
- 1 tsp. fresh parsley, chopped
- ¼ tsp Salt
- ¼ tsp pepper
- 2 cups spinach, fresh or frozen, washed and dried
- 6 buns or wraps of choice

Directions:

1. Preheat the oven to 400°F.

2. Peel and dice the beets into ¼-inch or smaller cubes, put them in a bowl, and coat the cubes with 1 tablespoon of olive oil and the onion powder.

3. Spread the beet cubes out across a baking pan and put the pan in the oven.

4. Roast the beets until they have softened, approximately 10-15 minutes. Take them out and set aside so the beets can cool down.

5. After the beets have cooled down, transfer them into a food processor and add the cooked chickpeas and quinoa, vinegar, garlic, parsley, and a pinch of pepper and salt.

6. Pulse the ingredients until everything is crumbly, around 30 seconds.

7. Use your palms to form the mixture into 6 equal-sized patties and place them in a small pan.

8. Put them in a freezer, up to 1 hour, until the patties feel firm to the touch.

9. Heat the remaining 1 tablespoon of olive oil in a skillet over medium-high heat and add the patties.

10. Cook them until they're browned on each side, about 4-6 minutes per side.

11. Store or serve the burgers with a handful of spinach, and if desired, on the bottom of the optional bun.

12. Top the burger with your sauce of choice.

Nutrition:

Calories 353, Total Fat 9.2g, Saturated Fat 1.5g, Cholesterol 0mg, Sodium 351mg, Total Carbohydrate 57.8g, Dietary Fiber 9g, Total Sugars 9.2g, Protein 13.9g, Vitamin D 0mcg, Calcium 103mg

Cilantro Lime Coleslaw

Preparation Time: 5 minutes
Cooking Time: 0 minutes
Servings: 5
Ingredients:

>Avocados, two
>Garlic, minced, one tablespoon
>Coleslaw, ready-made in a bag, fourteen ounces
>Cilantro, fresh leaves, one-quarter cup minced
>Salt, one half teaspoon
>Lime juice, two tablespoons
>Water, one quarter cup

Directions:

>Except for the slaw mix, put all of the ingredients that are listed into a blender. Blend these ingredients well until they are creamy and smooth.
>Mix the coleslaw mix in with this dressing and then toss it gently to mix it well.
>Keep the mixed coleslaw in the refrigerator until you are ready to serve.

Nutrition:

Calories 119
Fat 3
Carbs 3
Protein 3

Delicious Broccoli

Preparation Time: 15 minutes
Cooking Time: 15 minutes
Servings: 8
Ingredients:

> 2 oranges, sliced in half
> 1 lb. broccoli rabe
> 2 tablespoons sesame oil, toasted
> Salt and pepper to taste
> 1 tablespoon sesame seeds, toasted

Directions:

> Pour the oil into a pan over medium heat.
> Add the oranges and cook until caramelized.
> Transfer to a plate.
> Put the broccoli in the pan and cook for 8 minutes.
> Squeeze the oranges to release juice in a bowl.
> Stir in the oil, salt, and pepper.
> Coat the broccoli rabe with the mixture.
> Sprinkle seeds on top.

Nutrition:

Calories 432
Fat 1
Carbs 24
Protein 12

Spicy Peanut Soba Noodles

Preparation Time: 7 minutes
Cooking Time: 17 minutes
Servings: 1
Ingredients:

    5 ounces uncooked soba noodles
    ½ tablespoon low sodium soy sauce
    1 clove garlic, minced
    4 teaspoons water
    1 small head broccoli, cut into florets
    ½ cup carrot
    ¼ cup finely chopped scallions
    3 tablespoons peanut butter
    1 tablespoon honey
    1 teaspoon crushed red pepper flakes
    2 teaspoons vegetable oil
    4 ounces button mushrooms, discard stems
    3 tablespoons peanuts, dry roasted, unsalted

Directions:

Cook soba noodles following the directions on the package.

Add peanut butter, honey, water, soy sauce, garlic, and red pepper flakes. Whisk until well combined.

Place a skillet over medium heat. Add oil. When the oil is heated, add broccoli and sauté for a few minutes until crisp as well as tender.

Add mushrooms and sauté until the mushrooms are tender. Turn off the heat.

Add the sauce mixture and carrots and mix well.

Crush the peanuts by rolling with a rolling pin.

Divide the noodles into bowls. Pour sauce mixture over it. Sprinkle scallions and peanuts on top and serve.

Nutrition: Calories 512 Fat 11 Carbs 20 Protein 8

Portobello Burritos

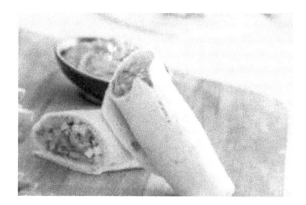

Preparation Time: 50 minutes

Cooking Time: 40 minutes

Serving: 4

Ingredients:

- 3 large portobello mushrooms

- 2 medium potatoes

- 4 tortilla wraps

- 1 medium avocado, pitted, peeled, diced

- ¾ cup salsa

- 1 tbsp. cilantro

- ½ tsp salt

- 1/3 cup water

- 1 tbsp. lime juice

- 1 tbsp. minced garlic

- ¼ cup teriyaki sauce

Directions:

1. Preheat the oven to 400°F.

2. Lightly oil a sheet pan with olive oil (or line with parchment paper) and set it aside.

3. Combine the water, lime juice, teriyaki, and garlic in a small bowl.

4. Slice the portobello mushrooms into thin slices and add these to the bowl. Allow the mushrooms to marinate thoroughly, for up to three hours.

5. Cut the potatoes into large matchsticks, like French fries. Sprinkle the fries with salt and then transfer them to the sheet pan. Place the fries in the oven and bake them until crisped and golden, around 30 minutes. Flip once halfway through for even cooking.

6. Heat a large frying pan over medium heat. Add the marinated mushroom slices with the remaining marinade to the pan. Cook until the

liquid has absorbed, around 10 minutes. Remove from heat.

7. Fill the tortillas with a heaping scoop of the mushrooms and a handful of the potato sticks. Top with salsa, sliced avocados, and cilantro before serving.

8. Serve right away, enjoy, or, store the tortillas, avocado, and mushrooms separately for later!

Nutrition:

Calories 391, Total Fat 14.9g, Saturated Fat 3.1g, Cholesterol 0mg, Sodium 1511mg, Total Carbohydrate 57g, Dietary Fiber 10.8g, Total Sugars 5.1g, Protein 11.2g, Vitamin D 0mcg, Calcium 85mg, Iron 3mg, Potassium 956mg

Mushroom Madness Stroganoff

Preparation Time: 30 minutes

Cooking Time: 25 minutes

Serving: 4

Ingredients:

- 2 cups gluten-free noodles
- 1 small onion, chopped
- 2 cups vegetable broth
- 2 tbsp. almond flour
- 1 tbsp. tamari
- 1 tsp. tomato paste
- 1 tsp. lemon juice
- 3 cups mushrooms, chopped
- 1 tsp. thyme
- 3 cups raw spinach
- 1 tbsp. apple cider vinegar
- 1 tbsp. olive oil
- ¼ tsp Salt
- ¼ tsp pepper

- 2 tbsp. fresh parsley

Directions:

1. Organize the noodles according to the package instructions.

2. Warmth the olive oil in a large skillet over medium heat.

3. Add the chopped onion and sauté until soft—for about 5 minutes.

4. Stir in the flour, vegetable broth, tamari, tomato paste, and lemon juice; cook for an additional 3 minutes.

5. Blend in the mushrooms, thyme, and salt to taste, then cover the skillet.

6. Cook until the mushrooms are tender, for about 7 minutes, and turn the heat down to low.

7. Add the cooked noodles, spinach, and vinegar to the pan and top the ingredients with salt and pepper to taste.

8. Cover the skillet again and let the flavors combine for another 8-10 minutes.

9. Serve immediately, topped with the optional parsley if desired, or, store and enjoy the stroganoff another day of the week!

Nutrition:

Calories 240, Total Fat 11.9g, Saturated Fat 1.3g, Cholesterol 0mg, Sodium 935mg, Total Carbohydrate 26.1g, Dietary Fiber 4.3g, Total Sugars 4.9g, Protein 9.9g, Vitamin D 189mcg, Calcium 71mg, Iron 4mg, Potassium 463mg

Moroccan Eggplant Stew

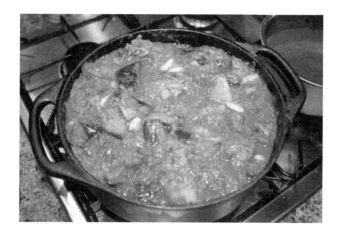

Preparation Time: 45 minutes

Cooking Time: 32 minutes

Serving: 4

Ingredients:

- 1 cup dry green lentils

- 1 cup dry chickpeas

- 1 tsp. olive oil

- 1 large sweet onion, chopped

- 1 medium green bell pepper, seeded, diced

- 1 large eggplant

- 1 cup vegetable broth

- ¾ cup tomato sauce

- ½ cup golden raisins

- 2 tbsp. turmeric

- 1 garlic clove, minced

- 1 tsp. cumin

- ½ tsp. allspice

- ¼ tsp. chili powder

- ¼ tsp Salt

- ¼ tsp pepper

Directions:

1. Warmth the olive oil in a medium-sized skillet over medium high heat.

2. Add the onions and cook until they begin to caramelize and soften, in 5-8 minutes.

3. Cut the eggplant into ½-inch eggplant cubes and add it to the skillet along with the bell pepper, cumin, allspice, garlic, and turmeric.

4. Stir the ingredients to combine everything evenly and heat for about 4 minutes; then add the vegetable broth and tomato sauce.

5. Cover the skillet, turn the heat down to low, and simmer the ingredients until the eggplant

feels tender, or for about 20 minutes. You should be able to insert a fork into the cubes easily.

6. Uncover and mix in the cooked chickpeas and green lentils, as well as the raisins and chili powder. Simmer the ingredients until all the flavors have melded together, or for about 3 minutes.

7. Store the stew for later, or, serve in a bowl, top with salt and pepper to taste, and enjoy!

Nutrition:

Calories 506, Total Fat 6g, Saturated Fat 0.8g, Cholesterol 0mg, Sodium 604mg, Total Carbohydrate 91.7g, Dietary Fiber 30.9g, Total Sugars 25.8g, Protein 26.7g, Vitamin D 0mcg, Calcium 133mg, Iron 10mg, Potassium 1714mg

Barbecued Greens & Grits

Preparation Time: 60 minutes

Cooking Time: 35 minutes

Serving: 4

Ingredients:

- 1 14-oz. package tempeh
- 3 cups vegetable broth
- 3 cups collard greens, chopped
- ½ cup BBQ sauce
- 1 cup gluten-free grits
- ¼ cup white onion, diced
- 2 tbsp. olive oil
- 2 garlic cloves, minced
- 1 tsp. salt

Directions:

1. Preheat the oven to 400°F.

2. Sliced the tempeh into thin slices and combine it with the BBQ sauce in a shallow baking dish. Set aside and let marinate for up to 3 hours.

3. Heat 1 tablespoon of olive oil in a frying pan over medium heat and then add the garlic and sauté until it is fragrant.

4. Add the collard greens and ½ teaspoon of salt and cook until the collards are wilted and dark. Remove the pan from the heat and set aside.

5. Cover the tempeh and BBQ sauce mixture with aluminum foil. Put the baking dish into the oven and bake the ingredients for 15 minutes. Reveal and continue to bake for another 10 minutes, until the tempeh is browned and crispy.

6. While the tempeh cooks, heat the remaining tablespoon of olive oil in the previously used frying pan over medium heat.

7. Cook the onions until brown and fragrant, around 10 minutes.

8. Pour in the vegetable broth, bring it to a boil; then turn the heat down to low.

9. Slowly whisk the grits into the simmering broth. Add the remaining ½ teaspoon of salt before covering the pan with a lid.

10. Let the ingredients simmer for about 8 minutes, until the grits are soft and creamy.

11. Serve the tempeh and collard greens on top of a bowl of grits and enjoy, or store for later!

Nutrition:

Calories 374, Total Fat 19.1g, Saturated Fat 3.5g, Cholesterol 0mg, Sodium 1519mg, Total Carbohydrate 31.1g, Dietary Fiber 2g, Total Sugars 9g, Protein 23.7g, Vitamin D 0mcg, Calcium 163mg, Iron 4mg, Potassium 645mg

Refined Ratatouille

Preparation Time: 90 minutes

Cooking Time: 1 hour

Serving: 2

Ingredients:

- 1 14-oz. block extra firm tofu, drained
- 2 large heirloom tomatoes
- 1 large eggplant
- 1 large zucchini
- 1 large sweet yellow onion, diced
- 1 cup chopped kale
- 1 cup tomato sauce
- 2 tbsp. olive oil
- 1 tbsp. minced garlic
- ¼ tsp. chili powder
- ¼ tsp. apple cider vinegar
- 1/8 tsp. fennel seeds
- ¼ tsp Salt
- ¼ tsp pepper
- 5 large basil leaves, finely chopped

Directions:

1. Preheat the oven to 350°F.

2. Lightly grease an 8x8" square dish with 1 tablespoon of olive oil and set it aside.

3. Combine the tomato sauce, vinegar, remaining 1 tablespoon of olive oil, garlic, fennel seeds, and chili powder in a large mixing bowl.

4. Pour the mixture into the baking dish and use a spoon to smear the ingredients out evenly across the dish's bottom.

5. Lay out the kale in one even layer on top of the mixture.

6. Vertically slice the tomatoes, eggplant, zucchini, and onion into thick, round discs; they should look like small plates or saucers.

7. Cut the tofu into thin slices, each similar in size to the vegetable discs for even cooking.

8. Layer the vegetable discs and tofu slices on top of the kale in the baking dish with an alternating pattern. For instance: tomato, eggplant, tofu, zucchini, squash, onion, repeat.

9. Fill up every inch of the pan with all the slices and stack them against the edge.

10. Put the baking dish into the oven and bake until the tomato sauce has thickened and the vegetable slices have softened, around 50 minutes to an hour.

11. Scoop the ratatouille into a bowl and garnish it with the chopped basil.

12. Serve and enjoy, or, store for another day!

Nutrition:

Calories 493, Total Fat 27g, Saturated Fat 3.2g, Cholesterol 0mg, Sodium 999mg, Total Carbohydrate 47g, Dietary Fiber 16.7g, Total Sugars 23g, Protein 29.1g, Vitamin D 0mcg, Calcium 498mg, Iron 7mg, Potassium 2324mg

Stuffed Indian Eggplant

Preparation Time: 90 minutes

Cooking Time: 21 minutes

Serving: 5

Ingredients:

- ½ cup dry black beans
- 6 medium eggplants, peeled
- 3 large roma tomatoes, diced
- 1 large purple onion, chopped
- 1 large yellow bell pepper, chopped
- 2 cups raw spinach
- 2 tbsp. olive oil
- 2 cloves garlic, minced
- 1 tbsp. tomato paste
- 1 tsp. coconut sugar
- 1 tsp. cumin
- 1 tsp. turmeric
- Salt and pepper to taste
- 2 tbsp. thyme, chopped

Directions:

1. Preheat the oven to 400°F.

2. Line a baking sheet or pan with parchment paper and set it aside.

3. Cut the peeled eggplants open across the top from one side to the other, being careful not to slice all the way through.

4. Sprinkle the inside of the cut eggplants with salt and wrap them in a paper towel to drain the excess water. This could take up to 30 minutes.

5. Place the eggplants on the baking sheet, and bake in the oven for 15 minutes. Remove the baking sheet from the oven and set it aside.

6. Heat 1 tablespoon of olive oil in a large skillet over medium-high heat. Add the chopped onions and sauté until soft, around 5 minutes.

7. Stir frequently, adding in the bell peppers and garlic. Cook the ingredients until the onions are translucent and peppers are tender, for about 15 minutes.

8. Season the spinach with sugar, cumin, turmeric, salt, and pepper.

9. Stir everything well to coat the ingredients evenly; then mix in the tomatoes, black beans, spinach, and tomato paste.

10. Heat everything for about 5 minutes, and then remove the skillet from the heat and set aside.

11. Stuff the eggplants with heaping scoops of the vegetable mixture. Sprinkle more salt and pepper to taste on top.

12. Drizzle the remaining 1 tablespoon of olive oil across the eggplants, return them to the oven, and bake until they shrivel and flatten—for 20-30 minutes.

13. Serve the eggplants, and if desired, garnish with the optional fresh thyme.

14. Enjoy right away, or, store to enjoy later!

Nutrition:

Calories 308, Total Fat 7.5g, Saturated Fat 1g, Cholesterol 0mg, Sodium 152mg, Total Carbohydrate 57g, Dietary Fiber 25.6g, Total Sugars 23.5g, Protein 11.9g, Vitamin D 0mcg, Calcium 134mg, Iron 5mg, Potassium 2027mg

Brown Basmati Rice Pilaf

Preparation Time: 10 minutes

Cooking Time: 3 minutes

Serving: 2

Ingredients:

- ½ tablespoon vegan butter
- ½ cup mushrooms, chopped
- ½ cup brown basmati rice
- 3 tablespoons water
- 1/8 teaspoon dried thyme
- Ground pepper to taste
- ½ tablespoon olive oil
- ¼ cup green onion, chopped
- 1 cup vegetable broth
- ¼ teaspoon salt
- ¼ cup chopped, toasted pecans

Directions:

1. Place a saucepan over medium-low heat. Add butter and oil.

2. When it melts, add mushrooms and cook until slightly tender.

3. Stir in the green onion and brown rice. Cook for 3 minutes. Stir constantly.

4. Stir in the broth, water, salt and thyme.

5. When it begins to boil, lower heat and cover with a lid. Simmer until rice is cooked. Add more water or broth if required.

6. Stir in the pecans and pepper.

7. Serve.

Nutrition:

Calories 256, Total Fat 8.8g, Saturated Fat 1.3g, Cholesterol 0mg, Sodium 318mg, Total Carbohydrate 39.8g, Dietary Fiber 1.6g, Total Sugars 1g, Protein 4.5g, Vitamin D 63mcg, Calcium 26mg, Iron 1mg, Potassium 144mg

Mediterranean Vegetable Mix

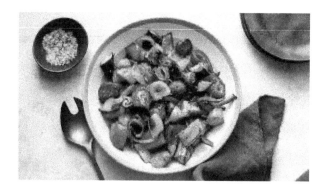

Preparation time: 15 minutes

Cooking time: 7 hours

Servings: 8

Ingredients:

- 1 zucchini
- 2 eggplants
- 2 red onion
- 4 potatoes
- 4 oz. asparagus
- 2 tablespoons olive oil
- 1 teaspoon ground black pepper
- 1 teaspoon paprika

- 1 teaspoon salt

- 1 tablespoon Mediterranean seasoning

- 1 teaspoon minced garlic

Directions:

1. Combine the olive oil, Mediterranean seasoning, salt, paprika, ground black pepper, and minced garlic.

2. Whisk the mixture well. Wash all the vegetables carefully.

3. Cut the zucchini, eggplants, and potatoes into the medium cubes. Cut the asparagus into 2 parts.

4. Then peel the onions and cut them into 4 parts. Toss all the vegetables in the slow cooker and sprinkle them with the spice mixture.

5. Close the slow cooker lid and cook the vegetable mix for 7 hours on LOW.

6. Serve the prepared vegetable mix hot. Enjoy!

Nutrition:

Calories 227,

Fat 3.9,

Fiber 9,

Carbs 44.88,

Protein 6

Fresh Dal

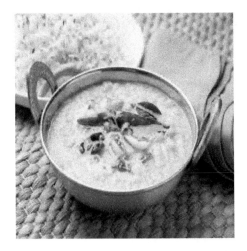

Preparation time: 15 minutes

Cooking time: 5 hours

Servings: 11

Ingredients:

- 1 teaspoon cumin

- 1 oz. mustard seeds

- 10 oz. lentils

- 1 teaspoon fennel seeds

- 7 cups water

- 6 oz. tomato, canned

- 4 oz. onion

- ½ teaspoon fresh ginger, grated

- 1 oz. bay leaf

- 1 teaspoon turmeric

- 1 teaspoon salt

- 2 cups rice

Directions:

1. Peel the onion. Chop the onion and tomatoes and place them in a slow cooker.

2. Combine the cumin, mustard seeds, and fennel seeds in a shallow bowl.

3. Add the bay leaf and mix. Sprinkle the vegetables in the slow cooker with the spice mixture.

4. Add salt, turmeric, and grated fresh ginger. Add rice and mix.

5. Add the lentils and water. Stir gently.

6. Then close the slow cooker lid and cook Dal for 5 hours on LOW.

7. When the dish is done, stir and transfer to serving plates. Enjoy!

Nutrition:

Calories: 102g,

Fat: 22g,

Carbs: 5g,

Protein: 34g,

Chickpeas Soup

Preparation time: 10 minutes

Cooking time: 4 hours

Servings: 6

Ingredients:

- 30 ounces canned chickpeas, drained

- 2 tablespoons mild curry powder

- 1 cup lentils, dry

- 1 sweet potato, cubed

- 15 ounces canned coconut milk

- 1 teaspoon ginger powder

- 1 teaspoon turmeric, ground

- A pinch of salt

- 6 cups veggie stock

- Black pepper to the taste

Directions:

1. Put chickpeas in your slow cooker.

2. Add lentils, sweet potato cubes, curry powder, ginger, turmeric, salt, pepper and stock.

3. Stir and then mix with coconut milk.

4. Stir again, cover and cook on High for 4 hours.

5. Ladle chickpeas soup into bowls and serve.

6. Enjoy!

Nutrition:

Calories: 302g,

Fat: 22g,

Carbs: 5g,

Protein: 34g,

Hot and Delicious Soup

Preparation time: 10 minutes

Cooking time: 8 hours

Servings: 4

Ingredients:

- 8 ounces canned bamboo shoots, drained and chopped
- 10 ounces' mushrooms, sliced
- 8 shiitake mushrooms, sliced
- 4 garlic cloves, minced
- 2 tablespoons ginger, grated
- 15 ounces extra firm tofu, pressed and cubed
- 2 tablespoons vegan bouillon
- 4 cups water
- 1 teaspoon sesame oil
- 2 tablespoons coconut aminos
- 1 teaspoon chili paste
- 1 and ½ cups peas

- 2 tablespoons rice wine vinegar

Directions:

1. Put the water in your slow cooker.

2. Add bamboo shoot, mushrooms, shiitake mushrooms, garlic, 1 tablespoon ginger, tofu, vegan bouillon, oil, aminos, chili paste, peas and vinegar.

3. Stir, cover and cook on Low for 8 hours.

4. Add the rest of the ginger, stir soup again, ladle into bowls and serve right away.

5. Enjoy!

Nutrition:

Calories: 102g,

Fat: 22g,

Carbs: 5g,

Protein: 34g,

Delicious Eggplant Salad

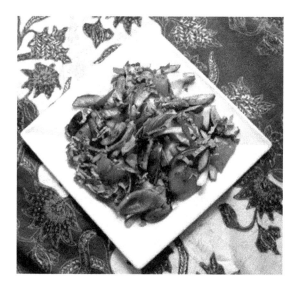

Preparation time: 10 minutes

Cooking time: 8 hours

Servings: 4

Ingredients:

- 1 big eggplant, cut into quarters and then sliced

- 25 ounces canned plum tomatoes

- 2 red bell peppers, chopped

- 1 red onion, sliced

- 2 teaspoons cumin, ground

- A pinch of sea salt

- Black pepper to the taste

- 1 teaspoon smoked paprika

- Juice of 1 lemon

Directions:

1. In your slow cooker, mix eggplant pieces with tomatoes, bell peppers, onion, cumin, salt, pepper, paprika and lemon juice, stir, cover and cook on Low for 8 hours.

2. Stir again, divide into bowls and serve cold.

3. Enjoy!

Nutrition:

Calories: 302g,

Fat: 22g,

Carbs: 5g,

Protein: 34g,

Tasty Black Beans Soup

Preparation time: 10 minutes

Cooking time: 6 hours

Servings: 6

Ingredients:

- 4 cups veggie stock
- 1 pound black beans, soaked overnight and drained
- 1 yellow onion, chopped
- 2 jalapenos, chopped
- 1 red bell pepper, chopped
- 1 cup tomatoes, chopped
- 4 garlic cloves, minced
- 1 tablespoon chili powder
- Black pepper to the taste
- 2 teaspoons cumin, ground
- A pinch of sea salt
- ½ teaspoon cayenne pepper

- 1 avocado, pitted, peeled and chopped

- ½ teaspoon sweet paprika

Directions:

1. Put the stock in your slow cooker.

2. Add beans, onion, jalapenos, bell pepper, tomatoes, garlic, chili powder, black pepper, salt, cumin, cayenne and paprika.

3. Stir, cover and cook on Low for 6 hours.

4. Blend soup using an immersion blender, ladle into bowls and serve with chopped avocado on top.

5. Enjoy!

Nutrition:

Calories: 202g,

Fat: 22g,

Carbs: 5g,

Protein: 34g,

Pumpkin Chili

Preparation time: 10 minutes

Cooking time: 8 hours

Servings: 6

Ingredients:

- 1 cup pumpkin, pureed

- 45 ounces canned black beans, drained

- 30 ounces canned tomatoes, chopped

- 1 yellow bell pepper, chopped

- 1 yellow onion, chopped

- ¼ teaspoon nutmeg, ground

- 1 teaspoon cinnamon powder

- 1 tablespoon chili powder

- 1 teaspoon cumin, ground

- 1/8 teaspoon cloves, ground

- A pinch of sea salt

- Black pepper to the taste

Directions:

1. Put pumpkin puree in your slow cooker.

2. Add black beans, tomatoes, onion, bell pepper, cumin, nutmeg, cinnamon, chili powder, cloves, salt and pepper, stir, cover and cook on Low for 8 hours.

3. Stir your chili again, divide into bowls and serve.

4. Enjoy!

Nutrition:

Calories: 242g,

Fat: 22g,

Carbs: 5g,

Protein: 34g,

Crazy Cauliflower and Zucchini Surprise

Preparation time: 10 minutes

Cooking time: 3 hours and 30 minutes

Servings: 4

Ingredients:

- 1 cauliflower head, florets separated
- 2 garlic cloves, minced
- ¾ cup red onion, chopped
- 1 teaspoon basil, dried
- 2 teaspoons oregano flakes
- 28 ounces canned tomatoes, chopped
- ¼ teaspoon red pepper flakes
- ½ cup veggie stock
- 5 zucchinis, cut with a spiralizer
- A pinch of salt
- Black pepper to the taste

Directions:

1. Put cauliflower florets in your slow cooker.

2. Add garlic, onion, basil, oregano, tomatoes, stock, pepper flakes, salt and pepper, stir, cover and cook on High for 3 hours and 30 minutes.

3. Mash cauliflower mix a bit using a potato masher.

4. Divide zucchini noodles in bowls, top each with cauliflower mix and serve.

5. Enjoy!

Nutrition:

Calories: 302g,

Fat: 22g,

Carbs: 5g,

Protein: 34g,

Quinoa and Veggies

Preparation time: 10 minutes

Cooking time: 4 hours

Servings: 4

Ingredients:

- 1 tablespoon olive oil

- 1 and ½ cups quinoa

- 3 cups veggie stock

- 1 yellow onion, chopped

- 1 carrot, chopped

- 1 sweet red pepper, chopped

- 1 cup green beans, chopped

- 2 garlic cloves, minced

- 1 teaspoon cilantro, chopped

- A pinch of salt

- Black pepper to the taste

Directions:

1. Put the stock in your slow cooker.

2. Add oil, quinoa, onion, carrot, sweet pepper, beans, cloves, salt and pepper, stir, cover and cook on Low for 4 hours.

3. Add cilantro, stir again, divide on plates and serve.

4. Enjoy!

Nutrition:

Calories: 302g,

Fat: 22g,

Carbs: 5g,

Protein: 34g,

Iron Abs Tabbouleh

Preparation Time: 15 minutes

Cooking Time: 10 minutes

Serving: 4

Ingredients

- 1 cup whole-wheat couscous
- 1 cup boiling water
- Zest and juice of 1 lemon
- 1 garlic clove, pressed
- Pinch of sea salt
- 1 tablespoon olive oil
- 2 cups canned chickpeas
- ½ cucumber
- 1 tomato
- 1 cup fresh parsley
- ¼ cup fresh mint
- 2 scallions
- 4 tablespoons sunflower seeds

Direction

1. Soak couscous with boiling water until all the grains are submerged. Cover. Set aside.

2. Put the lemon zest and juice in a large salad bowl, then stir in the garlic, salt, and the olive oil

3. Put the cucumber, chickpeas, tomato, parsley, mint, and scallions in the bowl, and toss them to coat with the dressing. Stir with fork

4. Stir in cooked couscous to the vegetables, and toss to combine.

5. Serve topped with the sunflower seeds

Nutrition

304 Calories

11g fat

10g Protein

Lasagna Fungo

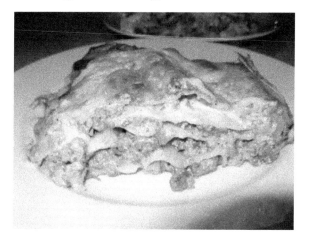

Preparation Time: 20 minutes

Cooking Time: 40 minutes

Serving: 8

Ingredients:

- 10 lasagna sheets
- 2 cups matchstick carrots
- 1 cup mushrooms, sliced
- 2 cups raw kale
- 1 14-oz. package extra firm tofu, drained
- 1 cup hummus
- ½ cup nutritional yeast

- 2 tbsp. Italian seasoning

- 1 tbsp. garlic powder

- 1 tbsp. olive oil

- 4 cups <u>marinara sauce</u>

- 1 tsp. salt

Directions:

1. Preheat the oven to 400°F.

2. Cook the lasagna noodles or sheets according to method.

3. Take a large frying pan, put it over medium heat, and add the olive oil.

4. Throw in the carrots, mushrooms, and half a teaspoon of salt; cook for 5 minutes.

5. Add the kale, sauté for another 3 minutes, and remove the pan from the heat.

6. Take a large bowl, crumble in the tofu, and set the bowl aside for now.

7. Take another bowl and add the hummus, nutritional yeast, Italian seasoning, garlic, and ½ teaspoon salt; mix everything.

8. Coat the bottom of an 8x8 baking dish with 1 cup of the marinara sauce.

9. Cover the sauce with a couple of the noodles or sheets, and top these with the tofu crumbles.

10. Add a layer of the vegetables on top of the tofu.

11. Continue to build up the lasagna by stacking layers of marinara sauce, noodles or sheets, tofu, and vegetables, and top it off with a cup of marinara sauce.

12. Cover the lasagna with aluminum foil, and bake in the oven for 20-25 minutes.

13. Take away the foil and put back in the oven for an additional 5 minutes.

14. Allow the lasagna to sit for 10 minutes before serving, or store for another day!

Nutrition:

Calories 491, Total Fat 13.1g, Saturated Fat 2.2g, Cholesterol 30mg, Sodium 959mg, Total Carbohydrate 73.5g, Dietary Fiber 9g, Total Sugars 13.3g, Protein 23.3g, Vitamin D 32mcg, Calcium 176mg, Iron 5mg, Potassium 903mg

Sweet and Sour Tofu

Preparation Time: 40 minutes

Cooking Time: 21 minutes

Serving: 4

Ingredients:

- 14-oz. package extra firm tofu, drained
- 2 tbsp. olive oil
- 1 large red bell pepper, pitted, chopped
- 1 medium white onion, diced
- 2 tbsp. minced garlic
- ½-inch minced ginger
- 1 cup pineapple chunks
- 1 tbsp. tomato paste
- 2 tbsp. rice vinegar
- 2 tbsp. low sodium soy sauce
- 1 tsp. cornstarch
- 1 tbsp. cane sugar
- ¼ tsp Salt
- ¼ tsp pepper

Directions:

1. whisk together the tomato paste, vinegar, soy sauce, cornstarch, and sugar in a bowl.

2. Cut the tofu into ¼-inch cubes, place in a medium bowl, and marinate in the soy sauce mixture until the tofu has absorbed the flavors (up to 3 hours).

3. Heat 1 tablespoon of the olive oil in a frying pan over medium-high heat.

4. Add the tofu chunks and half of the remaining marinade to the pan, leaving the rest for later.

5. Stir frequently until the tofu is cooked golden brown, approximately 10-12 minutes. Remove the tofu from the heat and set aside in a medium-sized bowl.

6. Add the other tablespoon of olive oil to the same pan, then the garlic and ginger; heat for about 1 minute.

7. Add in the peppers and onions. Mix until the vegetables have softened, about 5 minutes.

8. Pour the leftover marinade into the pan with the vegetables and heat until the sauce thickens while continuously stirring, around 4 minutes.

9. Add the pineapple chunks and tofu cubes to the pan while stirring and cook for 3 minutes.

10. Serve and enjoy right away, or, let the sweet and sour tofu cool down and store for later!

Nutrition:

Calories 290, Total Fat 16.9g, Saturated Fat 2.6g, Cholesterol 0mg, Sodium 512mg, Total Carbohydrate 19.5g, Dietary Fiber 3.3g, Total Sugars 9.1g, Protein 15.9g, Vitamin D 0mcg, Calcium 138mg, Iron 1mg, Potassium 434mg

Conclusion

In a nutshell, this cookbook offers you a world full of options to diversify your plant-based menu. People on this diet are usually seen struggling to choose between healthy food and flavor but, soon, they run out of the options. The selection of 250 recipes in this book is enough to adorn your dinner table with flavorsome, plant-based meals every day. Give each recipe a good read and try them out in the kitchen. You will experience tempting aromas and binding flavors every day.

The book is conceptualized with the idea of offering you a comprehensive view of a plant-based diet and how it can benefit the body. You may find the shift sudden, especially if you are a die-hard fan of non-vegetarian items. But you need not give up anything that you love. Eat everything in moderation.

The next step is to start experimenting with the different recipes in this book and see which ones are your favorites. Everyone has their favorite food, and you will surely find several of yours in this book. Start with breakfast and work your way through. You will be pleasantly surprised at how tasty a vegan meal really can be.

You will love reading this book, as it helps you to understand how revolutionary a plant-based diet can be. It will help you to make informed decisions as you move toward greater change for the greater good. What are you waiting for? Have you begun your journey on the path of the plant-based diet yet? If you haven't, do it now!

Now you have everything you need to get started making budget-friendly, healthy plant-based recipes. Just follow your basic shopping list and follow your meal plan to get started! It's easy to switch over to a plant-based diet if you have your meals planned out and temptation locked away. Don't forget to clean out your kitchen before starting, and you're sure to meet all your diet and health goals.

You need to plan if you are thinking about dieting. First, you can start slowly by just eating one meal a day, which is vegetarian and gradually increasing your number of vegetarian meals. Whenever you are struggling, ask your friend or family member to support you and keep you motivated. One important thing is also to be regularly accountable for not following the diet.

If dieting seems very important to you and you need to do it right, then it is recommended that you visit a professional such as a nutritionist or dietitian to discuss your dieting plan and optimizing it for the better.

No matter how much you want to lose weight, it is not advised that you decrease your calorie intake to an unhealthy level. Losing weight does not mean that you stop eating. It is done by carefully planning meals.

A plant-based diet is very easy once you get into it. At first, you will start to face a lot of difficulties, but if you start slowly, then you can face all the barriers and achieve your goal.

Swap out one unhealthy food item each week that you know is not helping you and put in its place one of the plant-based ingredients that you like. Then have some fun creating the many different recipes in this book. Find out what recipes you like the most so you can make them often and most of all; have some fun exploring all your recipe options.

Wish you good luck with the plant-based diet!

CPSIA information can be obtained
at www.ICGtesting.com
Printed in the USA
BVHW052029120421
604748BV00001B/117